LET'S TALK BABIES

An Experienced Pediatrician
Answers Common Parenting Questions

Featuring: Dr. L. Frank Bentley
with
Patti and Steve

Let's Talk BABIES   Paperback Edition

Edited by Bryson Walker

Front Cover Design by Leslie Walker

Photography by Jairo
featuring Jesica and Maia

Copyright and Published 2021 by Walkercrest
All Rights Reserved

ABOUT THE AUTHOR

Dr. L Frank Bentley is a well-respected and experienced pediatrician who began his career in 1977.

In 2012 he was given the award: "Doctor of the Year" by the Utah Medical Association.

In addition to caring for thousands of babies in his own clinic, Dr Bentley has helped educate fellow doctors all over world from South America to Russia and from Asia to Africa.

DISCLAIMER

Please remember, this presentation represents the information and opinions of the time period in which it was first recorded.

The discussion is only meant to be educational in nature and in no way replaces regular well-baby exams or medical attention when required.

TABLE OF CONTENTS

INTRODUCTION

Caring for your baby during the beginning of its life is a wonderful and joyful period. With the right information, you can be prepared for the many challenges as well as rewarding experiences that come with being a new parent.

This presentation comes from a recording of young parents who sat down with their pediatrician, Dr. L. Frank Bentley, and asked him many of the questions that you might have regarding caring for the needs of babies and toddlers.

The conversational nature of this presentation is easy to understand and follow.

Now let's join Dr. Bentley as he answers questions from parents Patti and Steve.

CHAPTER ONE

Fevers

Dr. Bentley: One of the biggest challenges parents of infants face is being able to accurately identify how they should take care of their children when they appear sick. For example, the most common question I get is: When should I call a doctor?

Patti: Dr. Bentley, we ask ourselves that all the time. How do we know when to call the doctor? What types of things should we call in about?

Dr. Bentley: I think that varies with every parent. Certainly a parent who has had several children will have a comfort level that is much greater than a parent going through it for the first time. Probably the most common symptom that will bring children into my office is fever.
A fever is something that is not normal. You know your baby is sick when it has a fever, and we can define fever, and we can talk about maybe how high it should be and when to be concerned.

A fever is always a sign that there's some infection whether it's trivial or not

Steve: What temperature is maybe the point to go to call the doctor? What's a safe zone and what's the danger zone? When do you actually call about a fever?

Dr. Bentley: Well first of all, in answering your question, I think you need to be sure that it's a legitimate fever. For example I saw a baby in the office today that came in because of a fever but actually had just been in a warm car and over bundled. By the time the baby got to the office there was no longer a fever. The baby wasn't sick. So an elevated temperature may not mean a fever, and so I think as you are trying to evaluate, "is my child sick?" you should take the temperature a couple of times and unwrap the baby and be sure that it is legitimate.

Steve: I've heard different things as to where to take the temperature. And maybe there's really only one best way to take the temperature.

Patti: Do you advise us to take the temperature ourselves at home?

Dr. Bentley: Absolutely. I think you should be very comfortable taking temperatures on your children; your babies. Not that you have to take them all the time every day, but I think certainly if your child is sick, feels like it has a fever, is not acting well, then that should be one of the first things that you do. That's certainly one of the first things that a doctor is going to want to know is, you know, "what's your child's temperature?"
Rectal temperature is the gold standard. There are a lot of newer ways of taking temperatures that are a lot easier. There are infrared ear thermometers that are wonderful. We have one and in a flash, less than two or three seconds, you can take a child's temperature.

Steve: Accurately?

Dr. Bentley: Very accurately. As long as the infrared beam is aimed right at the tympanic membrane. If it hits the side of the eardrum or the ear, then you're just measuring skin temperature and not body temperature. The fever strips you can get are not accurate at all, whatsoever; they are all over the place and I don't recommend those. Likewise the pacifiers that turn a different color are not accurate. Taking temperatures in other ways perhaps…

Steve: How about oral temperatures?

Dr. Bentley: Oral temperatures should only be taken in older children that won't bite the thermometer, so that's only appropriate in older, school-age and above. You asked, "What degree is a concern?" And that really is difficult because you might have a child that is very, very ill with a temperature of 101 or 102, and a child that is running around the house with 104 or 105. And everybody's temperature stat– you know the part of the brain that controls your temperature– works a little differently.

Some kids just don't have fevers to speak of, and if they have much of a fever at all it may be a big-time infection. Other kids at the drop of a hat they'll have this huge fever and it's just very trivial. So I would say anything over 102 and 103 is something you should sit up and take good notice of. And say, "Hey, where's this coming from?" And if it lasts... The other advice is if your child has a fever that is just starting, and your child is not terribly ill, my advice would be just to treat the fever and watch the child. Now your first time around with your first child you may not feel comfortable doing that but a lot of those fevers will pass and will go away, run their course. If it's really an infection it will declare itself.

Patti: You mentioned that we should treat the fever. How do you recommend treating a fever?

Dr. Bentley: There are several ways of treating a fever and probably the most highly recommended– and which I recommend – is Tylenol or acetaminophen of any brand. Most places have a generic brand of acetaminophen and they're all fine. There's doses according to age that you can look up on the package and at your Physician's office.

Besides that, everyone wants to know if they should bundle them up. You know, when you have a fever you may get chills and you want to be wrapped up. That's your natural instinct, but if you do that then that drives a fever up even higher. So I recommend giving some Tylenol, then taking the wraps off, then if the temperature doesn't respond within 45 minutes, then you might want to sponge with some lukewarm water, or just get the child's hair wet, or put them in a bathtub and then with a pitcher, run some water over the shoulders. And that's for a temperature that's high, 104, 105 something like that. And your goal would be to get it down to 102.

Just a comment, if you don't give the acetaminophen first, then the child is going to chill when you sponge them and it will drive the temperature right back up. That's how the body creates that extra fever and extra temperature is by chilling; all those muscles contracting, creating heat. So if you just start sponging them or take off the wraps then you'll drive the temperature actually higher.

Steve: Ok, can I ask when you say take off the wraps do you mean take the child down to just a diaper or some comfortable clothing?

Dr. Bentley: Nothing. A diaper for even less than that.

Steve: Okay.

Dr. Bentley: That's what we do in the hospital. That's probably one of the quicker ways of getting the temperature down. There is no inherent danger in having a fever. Fevers do not fry the brain or cook the kidneys or do damage to your body. Fevers are actually our friend, believe it or not. And it can create a lot of anxiety but they help the body to drive out the infection. Germs can only live in a narrow temperature range, when you exceed that and get a fever, that helps to kill those germs. So there is some reason to have a fever. Should we then treat a fever? I believe we should because I don't think the value of having fever is that great. I think the discomfort is greater than the value. So I believe in helping children be more comfortable.

Patti: When you're in doubt, Dr. Bentley, would you have us call to be sure rather than wait?

Dr. Bentley: Absolutely. I very much encourage all parents to have a good rapport and relationship with their physician and not be intimidated by calling. The answer that I give to the question: "When should I call the doctor?" is when you feel uncomfortable. Everybody's comfort level is different, therefore when you exceed your personal comfort level you should call; whenever that is, and it will change as you get experience as a parent.

CHAPTER TWO

Vomiting and Diarrhea

Steve: Dr. Bentley, let's talk a little bit about when our child throws up. I can remember several times from when he was just an infant and spitting up to it when he was apparently quite sick and then really throwing up. It's really worrisome for a parent to not know why the child is throwing up and not know what to do.

Patti: It seems like at times it's just volumes and you're really worried. What's the kind of rule of thumb with that?

Dr. Bentley: Excellent questions, I think it's all a matter of degree. And certainly I think all babies spit up, some much more than others. As a pediatrician I get concerned if an infant is throwing up with almost every feeding, that really concerns me. Usually a baby's not going to get enough nutrition – and there's usually a blockage or some anatomic reason, some problem if it is several times a day, almost every feeding. Whereas a baby that might do it once a week or every other day or once a month, you know, kind of infrequently. There's a lot of reasons for that, you know, if they ate real fast on a particular feeding or maybe you had a Mexican burrito the night before and you tried to breastfeed your baby and that didn't sit well; there are a lot of reasons that are not real serious.

Then if you take a child like you say that is really sick and it's just really throwing up and it comes out real forceful, it might come out of its nose, which by the way, is okay. The nose is connected to the mouth so if it comes out with any kind of force it will certainly come out of the nose too. As another rule of thumb is that any vomiting that is green is an obstruction or a blockage until proven otherwise. That should be alerted to a physician right away, or even a child should be taken to an emergency room particularly if the abdomen is swollen and hard and distended.
Steve: Can I ask at what age that can happen?
Dr. Bentley: Any age. There are certain blockages that are more common in infants and there are blockages that can occur later in life so at any age that can happen. Any real forceful active

vomiting that is green is a blockage until proven otherwise.

And then there is a concern about a child getting dehydrated if they throw up enough that is always a concern. You know if a child throws up only a time or two that's not going to create dehydration. But a child that is actively vomiting for hours on end could result in dehydration. Usually when a child gets the flu, they'll just wretch and wretch and wretch for a couple of hours sometimes. And it might get to the point where they are throwing up bile which is kind of green, and if you don't do anything just let their bowel rest, they'll just settle down and they won't be hungry, they won't be thirsty, they're still nauseated, they just want to sleep, they just want to kind of hang out, and let everything calm down. And then a little bit later, they might throw up again but you can start giving them fluids to replenish what they've lost.

When should you call the doctor on vomiting? If it's really forceful or if the child is in a lot of discomfort then I'd call.

Patti: What if there's diarrhea as well as vomiting? Is there more danger of dehydration then?

Dr. Bentley: Absolutely. If you're losing fluids out of both ends then they can get dehydrated in a big hurry, particularly with young babies. Under a year of age, they are susceptible to dehydration. It only takes a few hours of that. On the other hand, if a baby only has three or four diarrheal stools a day that's probably part and parcel of having the flu. It's all a matter of degree but those would be good rules of thumb.

Steve: Dr. Bentley, we've talked some about dehydration. Maybe you can help us understand the best way to help a child to not get dehydrated; to replenish those fluids that are being lost through illness or whatever.

Dr. Bentley: You have to realize Steve, anytime a child throws up it's not just fluid, it's also salt and potassium and some of these very important chemicals that we call electrolytes. They'll lose those out of their stomach and out of their bowels when they have diarrhea so in replenishing the fluid, you know you have to give them something wet, but it's better to give them something that has these salt and potassium and minerals in them. So examples of this would be Pedialyte, Gatorade, these commercially available electrolyte solutions with these chemicals and minerals in them. They are essential. As the child is losing, you have to replenish and it's best to replenish in small amounts very frequently. When it first actively starts vomiting, you wait for an hour or so, let everything settle down and rest, then try just half an ounce every half of an hour for a couple of times. Then maybe 2 oz every 2 hours, that could be a rule of thumb. That's how I personally would go about it but other physicians may have different ways. Just do small amounts and build up then they can tolerate it a lot better.

Steve: When do you actually give the baby a commercial product for the nausea, for the vomiting?

Dr. Bentley: My rule of thumb is that any child under the age of one to two you shouldn't give medication for vomiting or diarrhea. The reason for that is it will make things worse usually. They are very sedating often, they interfere with normal body functions, they can make obstructions and blockages worse, dramatically worse. You can throw a child that is mildly sick into a state of being severely ill. These medications are also associated with crib death. So especially under the age of a year you really want to avoid anti-vomiting medications.

Patti: That's great to know.

Steve: It really is.

Patti: Doctor, we were talking about bowel movements. Can you tell me what is going to be normal for an infant? What is a flag that there is a problem?

Dr. Bentley: I think that anything that is a departure from the child's own normal bowel movements, automatically is abnormal. As one of my professors said, "One person's diarrhea is another person's constipation." Every person has different consistencies of stools. Some people always have diarrhea, some people are always constipated.

I think severe constipation where a child withholds stools and goes once a week and builds up these terrible blockages is very abnormal. On the other hand a child that has diarrhea multiple times a day – and this is different from breast milk stools which can be 10 or 12 times a day, almost every feeding, and that's normal – but say a child is normally having a bowel movement a day and suddenly is having green diarrhea that is straight water running down the leg, that's all of a sudden abnormal.

Patti: So you become kind of familiar with what's normal, and when it's a departure, you would call.

Dr. Bentley: And I might add Patti, that a lot of people are concerned when their child's stool or diarrhea turns green. Well, what if you give the child a lot of green vegetables, or what if a child drinks green punch. I mean, there are a lot of normal reasons for green stools. So the green color by itself doesn't necessarily mean a whole lot. You can have a totally normal child that's having a green stool and you just look at it and say, yeah, it's green. But you can also have a child that is really sick and is pooping its brains out and it's green and you would be a lot more concerned.

Patti: I was told that if the diaper looks very mucousy that would be a problem. Is that right?

Dr. Bentley: That can be a problem Patti, but a lot of baby stools, again particularly if breastfed, or if they have a bad cold and they're swallowing mucus from being congested, they'll have mucousy stools. But, if a baby or a child is having really chronic diarrhea going on week after week and there's blood and there's mucus in the stool it usually means there's some infection, so yes that can be a danger sign.

CHAPTER THREE

The Croup, Hiccups and other Breathing Problems

Patti: What should we do if we see our baby having breathing problems?

Dr. Bentley: I think of all the urgencies or emergencies, breathing problems would rank right up there at the top of the list. It depends on how serious the breathing problem is. Patti, has your child ever had croup?

Patti: Now when you say croup are you referring to when they're having a deep heavy cough and where they're struggling to breathe? Am I correct, is that it?

Dr. Bentley: Croup actually is a brassy, dog-like, barky cough that comes on at night after the baby has gone to bed. It's associated with a cold, and their lungs get really tight and they have difficulty breathing. They have real difficulty moving air in and out.

Patti: And what would we do?

Dr. Bentley: If he's really pretty tight even after he's calmed down, I would take some outside advice; either calling the doctor or even going to the emergency room if it's more serious. But you should at least call the doctor to get advice on what to do during the rest of the night. Using a humidifier helps, and sometimes turning the shower on and steaming up the bathroom. You can have summertime croup and then you can open up a freezer compartment and have the baby breathe cold air coming out of the freezer.

Steve: There's humidifiers which I think are cold air and vaporizers which are warm air. Which of those are better?

Dr. Bentley: They're both equally effective; they both deliver good humidity; humidified air to the baby. The humidifier or cold air is safer than a vaporizer. Every year I treat several bad burns on kids that get into that boiling water in a vaporizer. I had one just last year that poured the whole thing down his front and had to be taken to a burn center. So that is a potential danger.

We don't feel that Vicks Vapor Rub and stuff like that that you would put in a vaporizer is that big of a help to advocate that you have a hot mist. The cool mist really is the safest. But going back to respiratory difficulties, it's kind of like having a fever. You can have a child with a big fever and not have a lot of difficulty. Then you can have a child that has a big cough and is playful, energetic, and not that sick, and although that is something that should be addressed in the doctor's office at some point, it's not necessarily something that you have to rush to the emergency room at night. On the other hand you can have a child that is not running a fever but is really struggling to breathe, and you don't know why, maybe a piece of a toy, maybe just a virus that's causing swelling in his throat, it might be asthma, it might be a variety of reasons and that's for the doctor to determine. What you know is that your baby is having difficulty breathing. And if your baby can't breathe, then your baby is having big time troubles.

Patti: When we first brought our daughter home from the hospital she seemed to have hiccups every couple hours. Is this normal? What should we do?

Dr. Bentley: It is normal. A lot of babies hiccup, and they hiccup a lot. It's not a sign of indigestion; it's not a sign of anything wrong with their stomach or their intestines. And you know what? Most babies who hiccup after they're born, were hiccuppers before they were born. And they bounced around inside that uterus for quite a while before they were born. That is fairly normal, and it doesn't hurt them and it's not uncomfortable for them. Do you know another thing that's normal with babies? Congestion. Babies are always congested for the first few months.

Patti: Newborn infants?

Dr. Bentley: Newborn babies.

Patti: How would you know the difference if it did become an actual cold?

Dr. Bentley: Well, with a cold, a baby wouldn't eat well, wouldn't feel well, would act pretty grumpy, would sleep excessively. All babies sleep a lot, but there would be more than what the baby is baseline sleeping. And there's a lot of difference between a baby that is a noisy breather and a baby that is having difficulty breathing; a baby that's kind of working hard to breathe is different than just kind of noisy. A noisy breather is normal.

CHAPTER FOUR

Jaundice

Steve: We were cautioned about jaundice and to check the baby's color right after it was newborn. Could you explain a little bit about jaundice to help us understand that?

Dr. Bentley: Jaundice is a yellow coloring that babies have. All babies are jaundiced to some degree or another; some are really daffodils. They are really yellow. Jaundice, without getting real technical, is part of the metabolism of the baby's liver. And the baby's liver has been dormant inside the mom. The mom's liver has been doing all that metabolism. The baby is born and cut off from the mom and so it's liver all of a sudden has to assume all that responsibility and it takes a few days for that to get geared up and to work. And so babies will get jaundice and that usually peaks about the third or fourth day of life. It will get better. Breastfed babies have more jaundice than non-breastfed babies.

Steve: What accounts for that?

Dr. Bentley: Breast milk has an action on the baby's liver that slows it down. There are some hormones in the breast milk. It's nothing serious, but it can last up to 6 weeks on a breastfed baby whereas in a bottle fed baby the jaundice will disappear after 5 to 7 Days.

Jaundice is only serious if it's really, really high. It can cause brain damage and can be really serious. So it's a matter of degree. That's why doctors that allow babies to go home really early in the first 24 hours of life will want to see them back in the office at about the third day of life to see if they're getting jaundiced. They will also answer a lot of other questions you may have. If the baby stays in the hospital the doctor and the nurses have a chance to evaluate the baby to see if it is getting more jaundiced and be tested if it's getting too high. But all babies are somewhat jaundiced and it's just a matter of degree.

Steve: What do you do to treat jaundice if it is of such a degree as needs treating?

Dr. Bentley: If it's too high, then special lights, fluorescent lights, are set up over the baby's crib and that changes the jaundice into something that the kidneys can take care of. Again, it depends on how high it is. If the jaundice is so high that even the lights won't take care of it then the babies are put in the hospital and special blood transfusions are given to lower it. But there are ways to take care of jaundice now.

Steve: What percentage of babies may need the lights, and how often is further treatment, the transfusion or hospitalization needed?

Dr. Bentley: Probably about 10 to 15% of babies will go under lights. Only in a rare circumstance would a baby need a blood transfusion.

CHAPTER FIVE

Runny Nose

Patti: Are runny noses a sign that something is wrong?

Dr. Bentley: Green runny noses are usually a sign of infection; so that can be a red flag. Now whether that needs to be treated or not, depends on if a child is otherwise doing great; not running a fever, remaining active, and it just barely started. If it's a green runny nose, then I'd probably watch it. But, a clear runny nose is usually not an infection, it's usually just a virus or early stages of a cold or maybe some allergies.

Again if it's really handicapping or interfering with the baby's ability to breathe or to nurse or to feed or to sleep, then you will want to talk to your doctor about treating it. It can be treated with either decongestants or if it's really turning green then the baby may have an infection and perhaps will need an antibiotic. So those are the rules of thumb that I have. Again, if it interferes with or creates some difficulty with the baby breathing then I get more concerned.

Patti: As a mother, should I trust my instincts when I think there is something that is wrong?

Dr. Bentley: You know what? I trust mom's instincts more than anything else. I trust them more than my own instincts many times. When parents come in and tell me they think their child is sick I believe them. They know. They know their child, they are with their child, they know every nuance, every subtlety and when something isn't right then that's up to me to find out why and where.

Patti: That's comforting to me as a parent.

Steve: It really is.

Dr. Bentley: Well Patti and Steve, we've talked a lot about different illnesses and conditions and when you call the doctor and is my child or baby sick? That's all very difficult to anticipate and to always know what to do and what's going to happen. I think when it's all said and done, you should call your doctor when you feel uncomfortable or concerned, no matter how trivial you think it might seem to your physician, it's important to you and should be important to your doctor and to his nurse.

You should also pick your physician such that you feel comfortable in calling. There should never be any intimidation, or your physician feeling estranged from his patients. I feel that physicians are the health consultant for the families they care for and should always be accessible.

CHAPTER SIX

Proper Nutrition

Dr. Bentley: You know one of the most important responsibilities that a parent has is to ensure that proper nutrition is given to their baby. This is absolutely essential to good health for your baby.

Steve: As we brought our newborn home from the hospital, one of the biggest questions we had was breastfeeding versus bottle feeding. Maybe you can talk about the benefits of each of those and help us understand that a little bit.

Dr. Bentley: I feel that breastfeeding is superior to any other way of providing nutrition to the baby. We don't know all the goodies that are in breast milk nor can we be so arrogant as to think we can totally duplicate breast milk in an artificial formula.

We are fortunate to have our babies in a day and age when there are some very good formulas. If Mom is unable, or for whatever reason breastfeeding doesn't work out, then there are some excellent formulas that will safely and healthily provide good nutrition for the baby.
It wasn't too long ago, as we look at history, that if a mom couldn't breastfeed her baby, 50% of babies died. That's incredible to think of that. They died from not getting proper nutrition, or what they were fed wasn't as effective, or it was spoiled, or there just wasn't the availability of a good alternative way to feed their babies. So therefore, breast is best, but not the only way. And I'm very supportive of whichever way the Mom feels like is the best way for her.

Patti: Do you have a preference of which formula you would recommend?

Dr. Bentley: I don't, and I feel that it is a parent's choice. There's a lot of good formulas. There's easily five or six that are very comparable. So rather than endorsing a specific brand let me just say that the dominant formulas that are available are all good. I don't know of any single formula right now that is a bad formula.

Of course we live in a time when you can do your own research online and read reviews.

CHAPTER SEVEN

Normal Size and Weight

Steve: Dr. Bentley, maybe you can tell us how much a baby should weigh. What is a normal birth weight?

Dr. Bentley: Well the average birth weight of a baby is about seven-and-a-half pounds. That of course varies with prematurity, with other medical conditions that the mom might have and certainly the sizes of the parents. These and other factors will all have an impact on how much babies weigh and how much they gain. Then, before babies start gaining, the interesting thing is that babies will lose about a half a pound during the first few days of life. Then they gain that as they start developing an appetite and the mother's milk comes in and they start eating more. So they'll regain that and they will get back to their birth weight by about a week of age and then will start gaining about an ounce a day after that.

Steve: Why do they lose that half pound or pound?

Dr. Bentley: That is usually just fluid that's in their body that they lose. It's not real weight loss because their birth weight is their weight plus a lot of fluid.

Patti: Our first child was a boy and he weighed ten pounds. Our second child is a girl and she weighed seven-and-a-half pounds. Did I do something to cause our first baby to be that big?

Dr. Bentley: Boy, a lot of chocolates in that first pregnancy!

(Patti and Steve laugh)

Dr. Bentley: No, there are a lot of reasons for a baby gaining a lot of weight. Certainly maternal diet might be part of that. If a mother has a tendency towards diabetes or another metabolic condition that can add to it. Every baby is different. Usually however, babies will get a little bigger with each pregnancy. So that's an unusual situation where the first baby is so much bigger than the second one.

Patti: Yeah, I did go over two weeks.

Dr. Bentley: On the first baby?

Patti: Yes. Two weeks longer.

Dr. Bentley: Yeah and that will– you expect a baby to gain about a pound per week, there are your two pounds if you went over two weeks.

Steve: Does gender have anything to do with weight?

Dr. Bentley: No. None. Boys don't necessarily weigh more than girls. I had a mother in the office today who wanted to know if boys are bigger. Her baby was this huge boy, but I'd just seen a girl who was even bigger than that boy earlier in the day.

Patti: Could you tell us what normal weight gain is?

Dr. Bentley: That is a very frequent concern of parents: Is my baby gaining weight? Because that implies that your baby is normal, that you are feeding your baby adequately, that you're being a good parent. We expect babies to gain about an ounce a day so that's about a pound every two weeks. Sometimes babies gain faster than that. But that's about 2 pounds a month. They usually double their birth weight by about 4 to 6 months of age. If a baby's average weight is 7 1/2 pounds at birth, they're usually 14 to 16 lbs by about 4 months of age and they triple it by the year mark. So usually they are about 21 or 22 lbs by a year of age and usually 30 lbs at 3 years of age. That's a rough measurement. Certainly if you are an NBA basketball player you are going to have a bigger child than that. Or if you are a jockey you are going to have a much smaller child than that but that's the average.

Steve: We've seen other people's kids, and of course our own are perfect! But we've seen other people's kids and sometimes you see a little chunky baby. Does that mean the parents are maybe not doing what they should be doing as far as nutrition goes?

Dr. Bentley: Well that may be normal for that baby. A baby is born with a certain body type. I think of it this way, when the egg is fertilized. We'll start from the beginning. When the egg is fertilized and the sperm and the egg unite, there is a genetic blueprint that is made. Okay, that tells all kinds of things. That tells the color of the eyes, the shape of the head, the shape of the nose. It also tells how big that baby is going to be. At two months, four months, even twenty years of age and so on. It tells how broad the shoulders are going to be, how big the wrists are going to be, how big the feet are going to be. That is set in stone. If I wanted to be a big giant I could not make myself to be a big giant. No matter how much I ate. It's not my mother's fault in the way she fed me that I'm not playing in the NFL. It's the genetic blueprint that I was given.

Now, if a baby is starved, abnormally, like in Ethiopia or something, then that can change somewhat and can vary the outcome, but say a baby is just fed normally, then you're going to have a variety of sizes and shapes at different stages.

You can look back in your baby book, it's a long answer for a simple question, but you can look back in your baby books and see that you were either skinny babies or fat babies and see your progression. And maybe your voice didn't change until you were 17 and you didn't start shaving until you were 20 or maybe you had a full beard when you were thirteen. All things like that are part of the genetic blueprint. So when you say, "Is my baby normal?" you have to take all of those things into consideration.

First of all, we go by statistical means; so studies done on tens of thousands of babies in our country tell us what is average. Then if we take two standard deviations from the average we can tell if a baby is fitting within what is considered to be statistically normal. But then you look at the parents, you look at what their childhood was like and then it all kind of fits together.

Now what about a baby that is really colicky, that is really fussy, that the only peace that mother gets is when she is nursing that baby. So she has that baby at her breast 24 hours a day and that baby just gets enormous. Well, in that instance that baby is fatter than it should be for behavioral reasons. That baby is being fed all the time. And there can be some kinds of abnormal things that can happen with children. If you reward children for good behavior by giving them a candy bar, then they'll probably be much heavier than they would be otherwise. Do you see what I mean? So, a fat baby usually, it follows, is normal, unless there are some other reasons, some behavioral reasons.

And that's part of what we do in the office is we kind of evaluate how things are going. "How's your baby?" we ask. And you can get an idea if all of that is normal in a pediatrician's exam. And if all of a sudden the baby's weight takes off for no good reason, then you kind of want to know. "Gosh, we want to know what's going on here!" Now some babies grow up and they really take off, and they have a big growth spurt, and you say, "Gosh, this baby is hungry every hour and it keeps me up all night long!" As far as you can tell your milk supply is normal and everything else is normal, but that's what happens with babies, they take off and then they'll kind of plateau in their growth. Everything will be kind of good for a week or two and then all of a sudden, bam! Things take off again. So those are also some variations on the theme.

That's a long answer to your question about overweight babies. Sometimes parents come in and think their baby is just emaciated. Of course if you look at the parents, maybe they are really slender people and you expect their baby to be more petite than parents that have much bigger body frames.

Patti: Dr. Bentley I've heard that a baby will keep the fat cells that it has. Is that true? Is that something we should be concerned about?

Dr. Bentley: That was a theory and a concern years ago. Probably to explain the occasional fat child that you see in a family of otherwise skinny people. Every once in a while you'll see a situation where a parent is concerned that a baby is too fat and they try to put them on a diet. That's really quite dangerous. Babies need quite a bit of fat as they grow. You say, "What good is fat? Fat is dangerous!" And we all shun fat like cancer. But fat really is very essential to the formation of nerves to the growth of the brain. Most of what the brain is made of is fat in certain forms. The formation of the sheaves around the nerves and the nerves themselves are actually forms of fat.

We believe that the growth and development of the brain and the intellect is stunted if babies don't get enough fat. Therefore the advice, in feeding babies, is that unless babies are breastfed is that they should be on regular formula which is all very carefully formulated to mimic breast milk and to provide enough fat and enough protein and enough other carbohydrates and vitamins until the baby is a year of age and then whole milk until 2 and then you can vary from that you can put the baby on other forms of milk whatever the family drinks, even skim milk, realizing the baby will probably eat a lot of other dairy products, cheese, cottage cheese and so on.

But to put children on diets is really dangerous. None of us have any idea what each individual child needs. You cannot unlock that genetic blueprint and pull out the recipe for how much a baby's diet should include at a certain age. A parent needs to rely on the baby's demands. If the baby acts hungry and requires a certain amount of food then you should give it. And not project your desire that you want to be skinny therefore your baby should be skinny at any particular age.

CHAPTER EIGHT

Crying

Steve: Maybe you can explain for us some of the common reasons why a baby might be crying.

Dr. Bentley: That's a good question Steve, I think probably the first and foremost is that crying is a way of communication for a baby. It is the way babies communicate with their surroundings and with their parents. Infants of course have no language, crying is their language. And so for a baby to cry is a very natural thing. It can express discomfort, it can express irritation at maybe being handled the way he or she may not appreciate being handled, being moved when he or she wants to stay in the position in which they were lying. I've always thought of it as a means of communication.

Steve: When our child was very young, many people thought and even our pediatrician thought that he had colic. And maybe you can talk a little bit about colic and what are the symptoms and what you do for colic.

Dr. Bently: Yeah the dreaded colic. Colic typically is infants about 2 or 3 weeks of age up to about three months of age. It's usually at night, a predictable time of the night. It lasts at least 2 or 3 hours in length. I think all babies are a little fussy earlier in the evening and that doesn't constitute colic. Colic is when a baby has a real full voice and lusty cry. It is inconsolable; hour on end, just lets you have it. And no matter what you do you can't interrupt or stop the crying.

Steve: We've tried some anti-gas drops. What's your feeling on maybe some of those treatments or some of those remedies.

Dr. Bentley: Well no one really knows what causes colic. We assume it has to do with abdominal pain or gas and so handsome there are some drops for gas that helps the baby assimilate the gas or pass the gas. And that seems to help some of the times and some of the times it doesn't.

Sometimes colic is related to the type of formula or maybe what the mother is eating. And sometimes it gets passed in the breast milk. Maybe it comes after a long hard day when a mom has been on the go and out shopping and hauling the baby around. Maybe it's quite hot, maybe there's been abrupt temperature changes. Maybe the baby's getting sick. There are a variety of reasons that would culminate in a baby crying.

I also think that colic is temperament dependent and somewhat temperament related. Some babies are pretty nervous, ancy babies. Other babies are mellow laid-back, do with me what you will type babies. And the real nervous babies, any little change in their environment, they are set off, they just go berserk. And other babies just roll with the punches. "You can give me a big huge ear infection and I won't cry a bit." So a lot of that is temperament related too.

Patti: We've been given advice like run the vacuum cleaner or lay the baby on top of the running clothes dryer to hear the vibrations. Have you found that those things have been helpful?

Dr. Bentley: It helps with certain babies in certain situations. It doesn't always help every time. I think warmth, vibrations, and motion will help. You may find that you can hold your baby in a certain position with a little bit of pressure on its abdomen and that seems to help. And again it might help one night and not help the next. It might help your baby and not your friend's baby. So it does help, sometimes, and there are devices that vibrate the crib and kind of give placental noises to mimic the environment from which a baby came. A lot of those things really do help.

A lot of people put a lot of mileage on their car during the first couple months of their baby's life. What else can you do to help settle a baby down? I think singing lullabies, recorded songs, motions and we talked about a lot of those other modalities. A lot of those do work and you just have to find out what helps your particular baby. Trial and error.

Patti: Dr. Bentley, what kinds of things should I look for when the baby's crying?

Dr. Bentley: That's a good question Patti. I think first of all you want to make sure that the baby's needs are taken care of, that the baby's not hungry. Check to be sure that he or she has been changed. Check little things like is the diaper pin sticking the baby? Or is there a hair wrapped around its toe?

Last year when a baby came into the office that had been crying, I found a burr from a plant or a weed stuck in its gum. And how it got in there you just never know. But you just look first and see if everything is okay.

Another common thing that often happens is babies will scratch their eyes. They kind of flail their arms around and in the process of doing that they can catch their eye with the corner of their fingernail and scratch the cornea. And that's very painful for several hours. It often clears up by the next day spontaneously without any other treatment, but that can often be the reason why a baby cries and will cry really hard for quite a while.

Steve: When do you say, "Hey, I've got to take the baby to the doctor?"

Dr. Bentley: I think that will vary with every parent and with the level of experience they have. Say we have 100 parents, and each parent has had a different experience and therefore different comfort levels, so that will vary. I will just preface my comments by saying that. But I think if you have checked all of the above things and the diaper and feedings and burping and all of that that I've mentioned, and the baby is consistently and persistently crying, and you're crying right along with it, then I think after two or three or four hours and you can't get the baby to settle down, then you should call.

And another thing I want to mention before I fully answer the question is, don't be afraid to just lay your baby down. Because I've known a lot of babies that don't like to be rocked and handled and massaged. They just want to be left alone to go to sleep. You know, "Get out of my hair I want to go to sleep." And they can't tell you, all they can do is cry. It's often very helpful to turn up the stereo, put the baby down, and walk out of there. Go take a little break. Then come back and see how the baby's doing.

Patti: Is there kind of a guideline? Ten minutes, a half hour?

Dr. Bentley: Time isn't as important I don't think as how the baby is crying. If the baby's crying is escalating and getting more and more violent or sobbing and just getting beyond the point of no return crying, then I think it's time to go in and pick the baby up and try to settle it down and start from ground zero. And certainly if you can tell if the baby is having periods of calmness, kind of settling down a little bit, and then starting to cry again, that's the kind of situation where if you don't walk in, that baby will learn to settle back down by itself.

I think babies cry for a lot of normal reasons we don't give them credit for. Usually parents think when they cry there is something wrong with their baby. A lot of what I do is reassure the parents, "Hey, maybe your baby just needs to cry or wants to cry." And that is very upsetting to a lot of parents to hear their baby cry. We're tuned into keeping our babies happy and satisfied. But there is a certain amount of crying in every baby's life.

The other point I like to make is that there is no limit to how much you should hold a baby or not hold a baby, I think it's very intuitive. You hold a baby when you want to hold a baby, and you put him down when you have to put him down. Your baby should learn to accommodate to your home and family, and not vice versa. In so many families, the baby is king and dominates the house and when he or she cries or spits up and everything then everyone else jumps up. And that is as it should be, they can't take care of their own problems. But I think they need to learn to adapt to their own environment.

Steve: What do you do when you set the baby down, and say you've got to do the dishes;and you set the baby down, and say he's been accustomed to being held for the last two hours, and he just starts screaming; major fit?

Dr. Bentley: Yes, he doesn't like being put down.

Steve: Yes, he's so accustomed to being held. On the one hand you say, "Let him cry it out." But on the other hand, he just won't stop! Just screams!

Dr. Bentley: Right. A typical scenario is you've just come back from vacation. You've been traveling in a car for fifteen hours a day for all week. He's been held by grandparents and aunts and uncles and you and everybody else who is not driving. And you get home and return to business as usual and you go to wash the dishes, you answer the phone or the door and you put him down and he doesn't want to be put down. He wants to be held, he's used to being held. Well, you still hold your baby when you need to hold your baby, you put your baby down when you need to put your baby down. You know, maybe you interrupt doing your dishes, you pick him up for a minute and settle him down, then you put him back down and you go back to doing the dishes. You can't hold him every minute of every day of your life, you'll never get anything done. And likewise, he wouldn't learn what it means to take care of his own discomfort or his own situation.

Patti: We were wanted when we had our baby immunized, that a certain type of crying or high-pitched screaming might indicate a problem. Could you tell us about that?

Dr. Bentley: That is a very good question Patti. I think different cries mean different things. Certainly with immunization a high-pitched, incessant cry that lasts for two or three hours or more can mean that the baby is having a reaction to the immunization and that should be reported to the physician.

I think parents get to know their baby's cry. If their baby is just annoyed, if their baby is hungry, if their baby just kind of wants company, if their baby is hurting, many times you come to know the pitch and tone and volume and urgency of your baby's cry. Sometimes you can be wrong. But the other thing I want to mention here is that a lot of times the parents say, "My baby's stomach hurts because my baby draws up its legs when it cries, therefore, I know that my baby's stomach hurts." All babies draw up their legs when they cry. That's what they do. That is just typical behavior. And it has no bearing on whether the stomach hurts or not. Yes, the stomach may hurt, but it may not be the source of the pain, so drawing up their knees just goes along with crying.

CHAPTER THREE

Sleep Habits

Steve: Let me ask a little about crying and how it relates to sleeping habits. We got into the bad habit initially of giving the baby a bottle to get him to sleep. And then of course if the bottle ran out or if he woke up in the middle of the night, he needed that other bottle to get back to sleep. And of course, at first we obliged and gave him the bottle. And when it came time to break that habit it was pretty difficult. When do you let the baby cry it out, as they say, and when do you try to console, pick him up, go for a ride, those kinds of things as it relates to sleeping?

Dr. Bentley: I've seen some really interesting situations. I had a family that would prepare about ten bottles, line them up on the window sill by the crib, just so they would have them right handy when that baby cried so they could go in and pop the bottle.

Babies can get very dependent on bottles, or rocking, or sucking their thumb, or breast feeding or pacifiers or all of the above to go to sleep. And if they don't have that, they can't go to sleep. Therefore, ideally, babies should be encouraged and trained to rely on their own abilities just to go to sleep.

So my advice, and what most pediatricians would say, is to feed your baby, breastfeed your baby or bottle feed your baby to satisfaction, and instead of having your baby be kind of dependent on always having something to go to sleep, you feed your baby until the eyes are starting to roll back and it's eyelids start to flutter, then you put the baby down. And the baby completes that process by itself, rather than having to go fully into a deep sleep. Because then what happens is if it moves, rolls over or gets awakened, then the stimulus or the pacification has to occur in order to get back to sleep.

Now in answer to your question of how long you should hold him and so on, the more you intervene, the more you perpetuate the dependency. And so the less you want to intervene.

But stopping cold turkey is very difficult, probably more cruel and unusual on the parent than it is on the baby probably, but it is very difficult on both. And most parents can't do that. I mean I can do it ater 8 or 9 kids, I can do it very easily, but boy I remember the first child or two is really hard; to walk out of there and listen to my baby cry, I just couldn't do it.

I find that if a baby is really getting that crying going and it's really getting to the sobbing stage, you know, you're in for hours of crying if you don't intervene and try getting the baby to settle down. Then you can put the baby down.

Steve: But you probably shouldn't put the baby down with the bottle or the pacifier.

Dr. Bentley: Exactly, or totally waiting until the baby is not crying anymore before putting him down. He'll start crying again, but you can kind of walk away from him and let him get used to it. I mean, that's all part of teaching and training your baby to go to sleep on its own.

Patti: Sometimes, you can go to a house and they will want it absolutely quiet cause the baby is in bed. Is this a bad habit? Can we turn on the radio? Can we have a normal life and conversation?

Dr. Bentley: Absolutely. However you train your baby, your baby will be accustomed to that. So if you tape your doorbell, don't allow visitors, have set nap times, nap times that are inviolate, your baby will get accustomed to that and will become dependent on that.

My personal preference is that babies are adjustable, they are malleable, they will sleep on the floor, they will sleep in the car, they will sleep over at your friend's house, they will sleep at the park, they will just be very cooperative. And you will have a normal lifestyle despite having children and a family. So go about your business, you baby will learn to adjust to that.

Now some babies, their nervous systems are just on the edge every minute of their waking lives. And so that kind of causes parents to do more, but even in situations like that I think you can still train them to be a lot more normal than a lot of people do.

Patti: That's comforting to know that we have a little bit of influence on how the baby will react.

CHAPTER TEN

Breath-holding

Steve: Dr. Bentley, when our child was quite young he would start to cry and instead of just going from one sob to the next, if you know what I mean, he would actually peak in crying and then not take a breath. And sometimes we'd say, you know, well surely he'll take a breath in a minute. It would go and go and go and it seemed like he was not taking a breath and we got kind of worried and would splash water on him to get him to take that next breath. But what do you do in those situations?

Dr. Bentley: That's called breath-holding and that can occur at any age including brand new babies. That is not an abnormal situation, but it is scary. It'll scare most parents to death when the babies hold their breath and turn purple and don't breathe. It can get so dramatic that even their eyes roll back and they'll even faint. Those are real dramatic breath-holding spells but will not likely harm the baby one bit. As a parent you need to be reassured by your physician that the baby is normal. I would certainly have the baby checked out and be reassured that you can let the baby cry.
My advice, as practical advice is when you can avoid having the baby crying then I would. If you're doing something and the baby is annoyed and starting to cry – say you're changing his diaper and he's starting to cry – instead of letting the baby get into a full cry and then try to intervene, pick him up before he really starts crying, settle him down, then set him back down and continue changing his diaper. That will happen to me in the office. I'll be checking a baby's ear and he'll start to cry and I'll know this is when he will start to hold his breath. Before he gets really going I'll just pick him back up and settle him down, get him calm again, then resume my exam. And then I can get through the exam okay.
Steve: Is there anything you can do when the baby is in the middle of one of those breath-holding spells. Like I say, we were advised at one point to maybe get water in your hand and splash the water in the baby's face and maybe that will help get the baby out of it. Is that okay? Maybe that's mean.
Dr. Bentley: No, it's not mean, and that is a very useful method

many times. A lot of times you don't have to do anything, and it will just naturally take its course. And even if a baby gets so dramatic that it passes out, the body's own mechanisms are protective and the baby will resume breathing and will be fine. It might be tired afterwards. But breath-holding is designed to scare parents I'm sure.

Steve: It works!

CHAPTER ELEVEN

Teething

Patti: Is there a lot of crying and discomfort involved when a baby teeths?

Dr. Bentley: Usually not Patti, but there can be. Some babies breeze through teething without a hitch and you hardly know they're cutting a tooth unless you look and feel a sharp edge, and other babies it seems that they really struggle with it. Again I think that is temperament related. You know, some babies struggle with everything. You know, they get a little cold and they're just really grumpy, Oscar the Grouch. Other babies can have a massive ear infection and hardly let you know about it. But my experience has been that teething is not all that it's cracked up to be, that it doesn't usually cause fevers, doesn't cause a lot of congestion, doesn't cause diarrhea, doesn't cause them to vomit, doesn't cause them to be sick or even real grumpy.

Steve: Now you say it doesn't usually cause any of those symptoms, but can it?

Dr. Bentley: There's no scientific evidence one way or the other.

Steve: Okay.

Dr. Bentley: And I think we all have anecdotal experience that might indicate that in a given situation it might. I think the danger in attributing a fever to teething, is you'd say, "Well, it's teething. And it's got a fever. So we don't have to do anything about it."

Steve: Chalk it up to teething.

Dr. Bentley: And I had one experience where a baby had meningitis, and when they finally brought the baby into the office and I said, "Gee, how come you've been watching this fever run so long?" And they said, "Well, we just thought he was teething." So I think it's better to look for a cause and ignore teething as a cause probably.

Patti: If it seems to be causing the baby pain, do some of the over-the-counter gels or remedies seem to be effective?

Dr. Bentley: They do, but they're very brief and last maybe just 15 to 20 minutes before they wear off. I think that one of the fever reducers or pain reducers like Tylenol or some form of acetaminophen that you give my mouth will be much longer lasting.

CHAPTER TWELVE

Ear Infections

Dr. Bentley: I get a lot of questions from parents saying, "My baby has been crying a lot, could my baby have an ear infection?" Have your babies had any?

Patti: Yes, many.

Steve: Yes, they've had some of the symptoms. In fact, we've noticed them rubbing or reaching for their ears.

Dr. Bentley: Ear infection has to be one of the most common causes of a baby crying. Almost always when a parent calls wanting to know why a baby is crying that comes up as a possibility.

I would say if a baby has had a cold, is real congested, a green runny nose and other respiratory symptoms and then starts really crying, and seems to be in a lot of pain, particularly if it is running a fever, I think you really have to assume it is an ear infection until proven otherwise.

On the other hand, out of the blue, if a baby has no other symptoms and is crying, even if it is kind of pawing at its ear, it may not and in fact usually doesn't indicate an ear infection. You may be surprised, but babies will start hanging onto their ears starting at about 4 or 5 months of age as a kind of a handhold; just because it's there and a handle, not because their ear hurts them.

Steve: She started doing that very thing.

Patti: She did.

Steve: And we wondered if she had an ear infection but there were no other symptoms, she seemed very content, she just reached for her ear.

Dr. Bentley: Often the babies will come in the office and we'll look at them and their ears are fine. They will often rub their eyes when they are tired for kind of the same reason. I would say that a baby that cries really hard and is sick, is an ear infection until proven otherwise.

CHAPTER THIRTEEN

Thumb Sucking

Patti: Dr. Bentley, our baby gets a lot of comfort from sucking her thumb. What are your feelings on that? Should we be trying to stop it? Can we stop it?

Dr. Bentley: I don't personally think you can stop a baby or child from sucking its thumb. I've tried over the years and there is no way that I know of successfully doing that. And everything I've read indicates the same thing. Not only that but there's evidence that shows in prenatal ultrasound reviews that fetuses suck their thumbs and their toes and their arms and they come out with hickies on their arms. So before they are even born they come out with that pattern and that habit. So that's very difficult to stop.

Your baby always has its thumb. It may not have its pacifier very handy but it already has its thumb. So it comes out already accustomed to that, it is really difficult to stop.

Now, can you teach your baby to suck its thumb? Yes. I've known some parents that wanted their baby to suck its thumb because they think it's cute. And so they will teach a baby to do that. I don't advocate that. But I think if your baby is really entrenched in thumbsucking there really isn't much you can do about it.

The only danger that I know of with thumbsucking is that it can affect the dentition. So you can create quite an overbite, or you can be looking at braces and quite an orthodontist bill later down the road. But that's the only real problem. Like a lot of childhood behaviors, the more attention you draw to it the more you entrench that behavior. So it may be best to just ignore it and let it take its course. Things that you paint on its thumb that taste awful...

Steve: Cayenne pepper.

Patti: I was told that you should try to put a sock over the baby's hands to not allow it to thumbsuck.

Dr. Bentley: I don't believe that any of this emotionally upsets babies, but I just don't think that it helps or it works. They'll just learn to suck around it or they'll suck their other thumb or they will take their sock off. I even put casts on baby's arms early in my career, I tried to do that. They find a way to rip that cast off eventually. They will chew it off and get to their thumb. So I just think you are in for the duration with thumbsucking.

Patti: What about a pacifier?

Dr. Bentley: I like pacifiers and I think babies have a real drive and an innate desire to suck; which is their instinct to get good nutrition I suppose. And if anything will intervene and get them to avoid thumbsucking it would be to get them hooked on a pacifier, and then you can always discard a pacifier whereas you can't get rid of the thumb.

Patti: So you might, early on, try the pacifier.

Dr. Bentley: Yes, that's a good idea.

CHAPTER FOURTEEN

Sleeping Positions

Steve: Dr. Bentley, we've talked a little about sleeping habits. Is there anything about sleeping positions relative to a baby's orthopaedic development?

Dr. Bentley: Babies, we believe now, should sleep on their back or their side. We believe they should sleep on a firm mattress and no pillow or down comforter or real soft type filling. Those all are found to be associated with or lead to crib death.

In terms of a baby's spine development, orthopaedic development, the only thing I can tell about that is that babies that are placed on a rigid board for example will have a flat head and will have some interesting spinal kind of defects that are created from that real flat, rigid board. But in terms of how we treat babies in our western civilization on just a mattress it should be fairly firm but not totally hard.

Patti: I've always heard that if you lay the baby on its back there is a risk of them choking if they spit up. Is that a concern?

Dr. Bentley: The only concern is with respect to premature babies. Maybe before they develop the gag reflex and can protect their own lungs by holding their breath and being able to choke and keep from aspirating. And it's really only the most premature babies, and when they are really sick, otherwise they should be on their back and side. In fact, studies are showing that in England for example, in Japan, in Scandinavia, they've really looked at the incidents of crib death with relation to how babies sleep, that the incidents at least double with babies that sleep on their stomach. And it is felt that their airway is somehow compromised and crimped; that maybe their temperature rises too high when they're on their stomach. But in terms of protecting their airway and keeping from aspirating when sleeping on their back, that's not a concern with full term, big healthy babies.

Steve: Can you change a child's habit? Once, for example, I recall when ours was about nine months old, she was sleeping on her tummy, and it was kind of a concern. But, of course, we couldn't force her or instruct her to sleep on her back. She had just sort of developed a habit of sleeping on her stomach.

Dr. Bentley: Right. At that age, they'll sleep anyway they want. They can roll over and crawl and they can get in whatever position they want. Initially, when you first bring your baby home, you put your baby down and that is where your baby stays. And when your baby gets to be 4 to 6 months of age then it's rolling over and assuming its own position.

Steve: So it's of less concern at that point.

Dr. Bentley: Right. You put your baby down and it goes wherever it wants. And the peak incidents of crib death is 3 to 4 months of age. So you really do have the responsibility of how a baby is positioned at that age.

Patti: How do you position a baby on its side? Would you use blankets?

Dr. Bentley: Right.

Patti: Is there a concern of the baby smothering by rolling around in the blankets?

Dr. Bentley: No, you would roll up receiving blankets and form a fairly firm, stiff roll at its back to keep it in its position on its side. You wouldn't want to pile up fluffy blankets or have something that it could potentially smother in.

CHAPTER FIFTEEN

Amount of Sleep

Steve: Tell us Dr. Bentley, how much should a baby sleep? And maybe how much at different stages should a baby sleep?

Dr. Bentley: That's a good question. That, just like how much a baby should eat varies so much with each baby. Let me underscore my answer by saying a baby will never become sleep deprived. A baby will always get whatever sleep it needs, whether it falls asleep in your arms, in a shopping cart or in your car. And I personally do not believe that the world revolves around the baby, but the baby needs to accommodate and adjust to its environment within the home. So doorbells that are taped and signs that say, "Shh, the baby is sleeping" implies that the baby is in charge and the world revolves around that baby. You know that probably also implies that it is a pretty grumpy baby that doesn't sleep that well. There are sleep requirements that I've seen that vary from just a few hours in a 24 hour period–I've seen as little as 4 hours in a 24 hour period–

Patti: Really?

Steve: Consistently?

Dr. Bentley: Yes. And as much as 18 hours in a 24 hour period of time.

Patti: In a newborn?

Dr. Bentley: In a newborn or even a little bit older. And as you think about adults, you can probably pick out people that you know that sleep very, very little. You know, there are stories that are told about Thomas Edison and people like that that only slept 2 or 3 hours in a night. And of course we all know people that need a lot of sleep. Myself included!

Patti: Oh, me too.

Dr. Bentley: That kind of underscores the answer, now the average is in between. Now about 20 percent of newborns will sleep 6 hours in a night without interruption. So that means that 80 percent don't. Most babies will sleep 3 or 4 hours then wake up for a feeding during the night. And so most babies will have at least one nighttime feeding, maybe two. But 20% of babies will sleep 6 hours through the night. You can look forward to having a baby that will sleep like that.

Patti: Can you try and train the baby to sleep through the night? Or should you always give them the feeding?

Dr. Bentley: There are a few things you can do to encourage a baby to sleep at night. I don't believe in training a baby until they're a little bit older, maybe 4 to 6 months of age. But what you can do is not pick up a baby and feed it unless that baby is truly hungry. For example, if that baby is sleeping right next to you at night and starts to move around a little bit it might go back to sleep. If you didn't pick it up. But that parent wakes right up and feeds the baby at the first little snort. And that kind of encourages the clock to be set at certain times.

The other thing the parent can do is feed the baby real frequently and regularly during the daytime and to not worry about people playing with the baby, holding the baby, other kids hauling the baby around the house, type of thing. I think that all can build up in helping to wear out the baby so it will sleep at night. Then by about 4 months of age that baby can be put out in another room or hallway or whatever; just a little bit of room away from the mother's bed so that it doesn't hear the mother making noises at night and the mother doesn't hear the baby making all those little sounds at night.

Then in terms of naps, most babies will take a couple of good 2 hour naps during the daytime so that it all adds up to 10, 12, 14, 16 hours of sleep during a 24 hour period of time with most babies.

Patti: Should the baby have its own room?

Dr. Bentley: I think so, eventually. Usually most parents will have the baby in their room just for ease of being able to pick the baby up and nurse or feed the baby during the nighttime. But I think as the baby gets a few months older and your comfort level with feeling that your baby is okay and breathing well through the night, those types of feelings, you can move the baby further away, into the closet or out into the hallway or across the bedroom and eventually into its own room; just depending on your comfort level.

Steve: How about as they get older but still under a year? What can you expect from their sleeping habits? When can you expect them to get a good, nice 8 hour's sleep?

Dr. Bentley: I would expect a baby by 6 months of age to be sleeping at least 8 hours a night. A lot aren't, but they should. And you can work on them at that age. What that means is letting the baby fuss during the nighttime hours. By that age they do not need a nighttime feeding. It may be programmed. It may be a part of their internal clock, but you can reset that internal clock by letting them fuss. That can be done progressively. You can let them fuss a little bit the first night, a little bit more the second night and a little bit more the third night and so on until that baby is finally sleeping. That can also be done by having more aggressive feedings during the daytime and keeping the baby more awake during the daytime type of thing. By six months of age you can really start working on a baby. A lot of parents do not feel comfortable doing that and so I don't force that on a parent. Certainly that has to come with their own comfort level.

CHAPTER SIXTEEN

Bathing and Hygiene

Dr. Bentley: Children's hygiene is extremely important to the baby's overall health, comfort and happiness.

Steve: Dr. Bentley, in bathing and in otherwise trying to provide good hygiene to my child, what are some good rules of thumb to go by?

Dr. Bentley: I like babies to be bathed everyday. I like babies that smell clean, that feel clean, that look clean.

Patti: Other people do too.

Dr. Bentley: Really. It's unreal how often you see babies that don't smell or look clean, but I like to bathe babies daily. Now some babies will have I guess real dry skin, real sensitive skin and so that may need to be adjusted and maybe bathe the baby every other day or maybe two or three times a week instead of every day.

That's also a very nice interactive time. It makes them bright-eyed and lively and they like to be bathed, and they are often up for the day and so you may want to bathe your baby in the morning. Other babies, giving them a bath kind of settles them down or winds them down and they will go down to sleep a little easier after a bath and so that might be an evening ritual that you should perform. You would want the bathroom warm. You would want the water not overly hot or warm but just skin temperature. And you would want to use baby soap or a real mild soap, not a typical hand soap which usually contains way too much perfume, and it is usually harsh. Some of the clear soaps are excellent for a baby's skin. The standard baby line of products that you are given at the hospital are the typical things used to bathe them with.

We do not recommend a lot of powders or lotions on a routine basis for babies. We feel that that plugs their pores and adds to many of the rashes that many of the babies might get; particularly if there is a family history of sensitive skin. So, just bathe your baby using soap sparingly and a little bit of baby shampoo and let that be it.

Patti: I've also heard that using powder, you can get it into their lungs and cause problems that way.

Dr. Bentley: That's correct. We get concerned about using a lot of powder. Now most baby powders are now made with a cornstarch base, and that's a lot safer than baby powders that used to be made from a talc base.

Steve: Let me ask another question about the temperature of the water. Is the shower water temperature that I like, too hot for a baby?

Dr. Bentley: Yes it is. You would want just above room temperature, their skin temperature. You would want what would almost be too cool for you in the shower because you can burn that sensitive skin of a baby really easily.

Patti: Really quickly. In fact we've heard that when you have a baby you should turn down your water thermostat.

Dr. Bentley: That's good advice. We've seen some bad, bad burns. In fact, babies die from scalding.

CHAPTER SEVENTEEN

The Soft Spot in the Head

Steve: What is the soft spot and how careful does a parent need to be in washing the baby?

Dr. Bentley: As the skull is forming and developing, that's just where the bones haven't quite joined together yet. And soft spots can vary from being very large, several inches across, to being just a little pin hole and still be normal. There is incredible variation. Soft spots are very resilient to pressure, to being handled. They're very leathery. There's no real danger in injuring the brain through the soft spot. So a parent does not have to be particularly careful in washing the hair or handling the baby or anything like that. You cannot puncture the brain by pushing on the soft spot.

Steve: We had occasion to become acquainted with a couple who had a child that ended up having water on the brain. Our understanding was that that was able to be detected by observing the soft spot.

Dr. Bentley: Sure, that's very correct. Water on the brain or anything that can lead to extra pressure on the brain can be detected if the soft spot is still open by bulging of the soft spot, that's a very helpful thing with physicians. We can feel the soft spot to determine if the baby is running a high fever and we're concerned that maybe there is meningitis. We will feel the soft spot and see if it is bulging or maybe under pressure. Likewise if the baby may be dehydrated, the soft spot might be retracted and sunken in more than normal. It is actually a little window to the brain and can demonstrate pressure.

Steve: How often, Dr. Bentley, do you find children who have water on the brain where they need surgery or other treatment for that?

Dr. Bentley: Water on the brain or hydrocephalus is a pretty uncommon or rare condition that certainly happens but is not a real frequent occurrence. Usually it is associated with other problems like extreme prematurity where babies have suffered perhaps hemorrhages in their brain thereby clogging up the reabsortive mechanisms of fluid surrounding the brain and that leads to extra fluid and hydrocephalus. Babies that are born with a defect of absorption of that fluid are really rare.

Patti and Steve: Okay.

Dr. Bentley: One of the things that always needs to be done at each well child visit to the pediatrician is measuring of the head. That, along with a careful feeling of the soft spot and measuring the head; plotting against the growth of the baby can tell you if a baby is growing too fast.

CHAPTER EIGHTEEN

Well-Baby Visits

Patti: When we bring our child in for a well-baby visit, what exactly are you looking for?

Dr. Bentley: We do a very thorough exam, quite quickly as a matter of fact. A pediatrician sees babies all day long and so even from the outset we can tell if a baby is normal or not normal just by how he or she looks.

We look at the size, how much weight and how much a baby has grown in length and if that is compatible with the parents and what we would expect from the baby's body type. We check the head measurement. Probably the first thing the pediatrician will do is examine the heart; listen for murmurs, listen for other heart sounds; listen to the lungs. And then we'll carefully examine other things. At first, we might examine things for why the baby might start fussing.

We palpate the abdomen. We check the liver, kidneys, spleen, other organs and for other lumps or bumps. We check for abnormal feelings or tenderness the baby might have in the abdomen. We feel a baby's hips and examine those very carefully, especially in the first year of life before a baby has started to walk because that can give an indication of hip dislocation. That is extremely important, it can run in families, it can be associated with cesarean deliveries or breech presentations of babies.

We examine genitalia. We examine, of course, the head, soft spot, ears, eyes, you know, we do everything we can to examine everything externally possible.

Most of the time the baby is doing well and the pediatrician will say, "Yeah, everything is going well." But there can be a lot of questions and a lot of reassurance to know that everything is going well. Pediatricians have occasion to see hundreds of thousands of normal babies. Whereas this may be your only experience for the pediatrician to see your child and so you need that input. Yes, this child is growing well and meeting milestones and having questions answered about their progress.

Patti: I know of an occasion where they had no idea about a problem. The pediatrician felt the baby's tummy and found a tumor.

Dr. Bentley: Right.

Patti: And that's something that a parent would not have caught until the symptoms got worse.

Dr. Bentley: I've had that experience. Or a pediatrician might find a hernia that the parents weren't aware of or a heart murmur, or an orthopaedic problem.

Steve: Yeah, my sister-in-law had a dislocated hip I guess and they had to do surgery at three months to correct that.

Dr. Bentley: That's a very important part of a physical exam.

CHAPTER NINETEEN

Shape of the Head

Steve: Maybe you can tell us, Dr. Bentley, what a newborn baby ought to look like. And I guess one of the things that I'm thinking of is really what their head should look like.

Dr. Bentley: Well, first of all, if a baby is born vaginally, the head is quite misshapen and looks like a conehead as it is squeezed and comes through the birth canal. There is often some bruising that is toward the back of the head which can be what we call a carput, which goes away in a day or so, and that's just a swelling of the scalp around where the cone is. That very quickly goes back to normal. A baby's head is very flexible and the bones are not joined together at all. They are free floating and so that goes right back to its normal shape within just a couple of days.

There can be a cephalohematoma which is a big, huge bruise on one side or even both; a big soft, squishy area on the side of the head. And that's where the scalp has maybe hemorrhaged and you have a blood vessel that has maybe bled into the space beneath the scalp and it gives almost like two horns in the back that are kind of soft and squishy. Those kind of solidify and can remain there, but then they eventually remodel and go away. But that is often a real concern of new parents.

The head also can have some other peculiar appearances that may be abnormal, especially as the baby grows during the first few months of life. As I mentioned, the bones are not normally joined together, but if they join together too soon, then you can have a baby that might have an abnormally prominent forehead, or might be too long from front to back or too skinny in the sides, or too wide and too narrow from front to back. You know what I mean? It just isn't round.

Maybe the baby might lie on its side, on one side preferentially, like if a parent always lies the baby down on one side in a crib. A parent might consider varying that position. Babies are very social creatures. They like to lie on their side and look out at the world that's going on around them. So a parent might change the position of the baby in the crib.

Steve: Which side the head is on.

Dr. Bentley: Exactly. Instead of always putting the baby down on the same end of the crib, you know, varying the position so that it will look out and take turns lying on different sides of the head.

Patti: If that happens to a severe degree, can that be an indication that the baby is being left too much just to lie in the crib?

Dr. Bentley: Right, or that the baby is being put in that same position too much. But you're also right that if a baby is being neglected and being left to lie alone, a pediatrician can kind of pick up on that. There are other cues. A baby may not be as social or may not be as responsive and be kind of withdrawn.

CHAPTER TWENTY

Hormones and Genitalia

Patti: Our son had enlarged breasts when he was born. What was that?

Dr. Bentley: That's a response to your hormones. As your body is trying to produce milk and your breasts are undergoing change, those same hormones are actually having an effect on him.

Boy babies and girl babies will both have enlarged breasts. Some will and some won't, but they may have enlarged breasts and may actually produce milk during the first few weeks of life. That goes away as the effect of the prolactin or your milk-producing hormone diminishes on the baby, but that is normal.

What can happen with girls is they can have quite a bit of vaginal discharge, they can have a little white milky discharge that's normal, again that is in response to your hormones, and they can bleed vaginally. They can actually have some withdrawal bleeding, or a period, a menstrual period as a result of being separated from the effect of your hormones. Of course that is just a temporary thing and then that goes away and then they are normal.

Infant girls are not having pubertal development at that stage.

Steve: What about other changes in boys? For example, our little boy, in addition to enlarged breasts, it seems like his genitalia was enlarged.

Dr. Bentley: That probably was not a response to maternal hormones. It may be that he had what's known as a hydrocele, which is fluid around the testicles and it makes the scrotum look bigger. That's very common and very normal.

It can indicate a hernia if it persists. We expect that that fluid will go away by about 4 to 6 weeks of age and if it persists then the baby has hernia. If it goes away, then that is an entirely normal event.

CHAPTER TWENTY-ONE

Birthmarks and Birth Defects

Patti: What about the little red patches on their eye or on the back of the neck?

Dr. Bentley: That's where the stork brings the baby, right? Those are kind of called stork bites. It's a traditional name. Those are little birthmarks on the face. Often there will be little marks between the eyes or on the eyelids or around the nostrils or the upper lip. Those usually go away, they usually fade. On the back of the neck, those are permanent. Those stay and almost everybody has one of those. If you can lift up your hair and look through your hairline, you can usually find some discoloration on almost everybody.

Patti: It seems like when they cry they get brighter.

Dr. Bentley: Right. Newborn skin is quite transparent and so those are real visible at first, and then as they mature and their skin gets thicker then those go away. Often it takes two or three years of life.

Steve: What are they caused from?

Dr. Bentley: There's no cause to be concerned about and the old myths that the mother ate a lot of strawberries or put pressure on the baby or anything like that are not true. They are not caused by anything harmful.

Steve: How about other skin conditions? For example, some little babies have what looks like pimples.

Dr. Bentley: Right. And newborn acne is a real thing. Usually it's just activation of the skin glands of babies being born and the skin is now exposed to air and that whole process of it now having to create its own oil and so on. They will have acne. Sometimes it can get infected and sometimes it can be quite severe so a real severe case of acne does need to be seen by your physician. But all newborns have some little rashes that come and go and move around and that is all part of being a newborn. Just as you are ready to show your baby at about a month of age the skin rash will be at its absolute worst! Mark my words.

Steve: How do you treat it? What should you do as parents when you first–?

Dr. Bentley: Nothing. You know, the only concern is if it is really severe, big pustules, you know, big zits. If they are really what you think are abnormal then you should consult your physician because once in a while those can get infected. But, don't pick them, don't macerate your child's skin trying to get rid of them.

Patti: What are some other birthmarks that we need to be concerned about?

Dr. Bentley: There are two significant birth marks that babies can have. One that causes concern could be a real dark birthmark, particularly if there's hair in it and particularly if it's big. These are called nevus and these are related to moles like you or I might have later in life. But babies can have these types of moles at birth and they can be very sizable. It can be several inches in size and it can be hairy. Those have the potential of forming skin cancer by seven to eight years of age or later and do need to be removed by plastic surgeons at some point in early childhood.

Another type of birthmark is called a hemangioma. And these start out as kind of purplish, somewhat raised birthmarks that can be anyplace. It can be on their face, it can be on their arms, hands, legs, wherever. And they usually will grow and get bigger and then they go away by about two or three years of age. The significance of those is that nothing usually needs to be done; no surgery, nothing, unless they are bleeding or unless they get infected or unless they are creating a problem like being next to an eye or some vital structure then sometimes they need to be operated on with a laser. But they usually will go away by themselves, and they will scar worse with surgery than if they are left alone.

Steve: What is cradle cap and how do you treat it?

Dr. Bentley: Cradle cap is kind of a golden, crusty build up on the scalp of a newborn. The medical term is ceborhia and a lot of adults have ceborhia, it is hereditary. The way it's treated is just with vigorous brushing with a very soft brush or even a toothbrush when you wash the baby's hair. My preference is babies should have their hair washed every day. If you ask ten pediatricians how often you should wash the baby's hair you'll get ten different answers. "Once a week, once every other day," and so on. But I like a baby's hair being washed daily. If there is a real problem with cradle cap then I recommend a dandruff shampoo that will take care of it along with a fairly vigorous brushing. That should take care of the scales and the build up that is on the baby's scalp. Actually, cradle cap can be in the eyebrows as well. You can sometimes see some little flaky build up in the eyebrows and between the eyebrows.

Patti: I've heard you can use baby oil to comb through it.

Dr. Bentley: Baby oil is often used, but it just serves as a lubricant to help get it off with a brush. It helps to grease it down so it's not as visible. But baby oil by itself is not a treatment for cradle cap.

Steve: What about birth defects in general? What is the likelihood of having a child born with a birth defect and maybe what are some of the more common ones that parents see?

Dr. Bentley: The likelihood is about 1 in 200 for some kind of birth defect. Some of the more common ones would be: cleft lip or cleft palate, and that is strongly familial, running in family lines; heart problems like heart murmurs, problems inside the heart, which are picked up usually pretty early, usually in the first exams that are done on the baby; other problems for example, six toes, or joined fingers or toes, or sometimes missing extremities. There are a variety of defects that way that can be pretty easily noticed.

CHAPTER TWENTY-TWO

Eyes, Ears and Nose

Steve: What are they seeing? And when do they start focusing? Or is there really any way to know that?

Dr. Bentley: You know, I've never had a baby tell me what it sees. It's hard to know what a baby sees. I think pioneers in the field of infant vision can kind of extrapolate from brainwave studies, but we believe they can see rough shapes, they can see light and dark, they can see bright colors. I don't think their cones and rods in their eyes are really well developed at first. Maybe the rods before the cones so they can see black and white and big shapes, and light and dark before they can see color. So we believe that their vision is quite rough and quite gross at first and just real close, near-sighted. So a newborn might be able to see 6 inches away, but not be able to discriminate shapes across the room. Whereas at about a month of age, they might see much like you and I see; colors and shapes across the room.

Patti: Is it true that all newborns are born with blue eyes and then they change?

Dr. Bentley: All newborn's eyes are kind of a dark greyish blue, a non-specific color, and it isn't until a baby is about four months of age that you can tell the coloration of the eyes.

Patti: What is the newborn's hearing like?

Dr. Bentley: We think they can hear right away. Think about some of the incredible changes babies go through. In uteral, babies are in a total, liquid medium. It's totally dark. They may have heard sounds, but it's through the uterus and through amniotic fluid. They have never breathed before. They have never heard their voice before. They have never heard sounds like you and I hear. They have never swallowed. They have never been touched. They have never been stretched out.

It is such an incredible change in their world to all of a sudden be born and be breathing air. Their skin dries out. They open their eyes. All of a sudden they are out of this dark cave. They are seeing light and seeing things move. They are being touched. And it is no wonder that sometimes babies are really irritable and grumpy and it is because of these big changes in their life.

We do know they can hear though and right away. And often, that is testable within the first few days of life.   For example, if someone has hearing loss in their family, if a sister, brother, cousin, mother or father was born with hearing loss, then the baby should be tested soon, to see if their hearing is intact or not. And a lot of hospitals have the ability to test their babies while they are still there after just being born. They put little pasties on their scalps and test their brain waves while different sounds are being presented to their ears. And they can tell if their hearing is normal or not.

We believe their smelling is intact. Studies have been done with different perfumes and they can associate right away what their mother smells like and the mother is the source of their food and who has been carrying them for all of this time. And they can tell, within the first few days of life, the baby can discriminate smells associated with their mother as opposed to smells from someone else.

CHAPTER TWENTY-THREE

Changes and Milestones

Dr. Bentley: Babies are all different and will develop at different rates. Parents must realize some of the changes and milestones of development to watch for.

Patti: Dr. Bentley, can you tell us some of the important milestones of our baby's first year?

Dr. Bentley: These are some of the things that we look at to make sure that babies are meeting their developmental milestones and which you can look to with a lot of pride and expectations and a lot of fun. The first real milestone is when the baby smiles. Babies start smiling intentionally at about a month to six weeks of age. You know, when you smile at your baby and it smiles back.

A baby will smile within the first few hours of life but it's not an intentional smiling. It may be when it is going to sleep or in a deep sleep or with a bottle or something, but not a social response like a little bit later that comes at about a month to six weeks. And boy that just opens your heart when you smile and your baby smiles back at you and not just because of a gas bubble or something. When you smile at your baby and your baby smiles back, there is instant bonding. I'll tell you that is love.

And then babies will start rolling over at about three or four months of age. They roll to their side first. Sometimes babies like to be on their back and not on their stomach and so they don't like to roll over to their stomach and so that's okay. Rolling from their back to their stomach occurs later, around 5 to 6 months.

They don't sit up until they are strong enough to support themselves and that doesn't usually occur until they are crawling around 8 or 9 months of age. So in between when they're rolling and sitting up and crawling, they are starting to scoot around. You put them in a crib in one position and you come back in and they are way over in the other corner. And they have scooted themselves around by their heels or on their backs or they inchwormed their way around. Sometimes they kind of lobster crawl or crab crawl or even do the army low crawl; different kinds of variations around that age.

Around 3 or 4 months of age, babies will start reaching for things.

So you can start putting something brightly-colored or shiny, kind of just out of reach and they will start to grasp for it. And then around 4 months of age they will actually grab it and bring it to their mouth. They start to drool and demonstrate other oral characteristics. Everything goes to their mouth, their fists, their feet, their toes; everything goes to their mouth at that age. Some will say, "That's teething." But teeth usually don't come through for a few more months. We believe that's just instinctive behavior on the part of the baby, it's just the oral phase. Probably so that they will be sure to get enough to eat.

Then babies are sitting up and crawling around at 8 to 9 months. They'll crawl to something and pull themselves up to stand. They will walk while holding on to a chair or couch and then climb up on that chair. Then nothing is safe! And you have to be sure that all of your dangerous items are tucked away and locked out of reach. And then of course they stand alone, will let go of whatever they are holding onto, and collapse to the floor. Big applause from the parents. And then they may take a step or two around a year of age. And that varies anywhere, you know, from the earliest I've seen is steps at 6 months and the latest is 18 months. And these are normal kids. So a really wide range of normal. And that is really important to emphasize, the baby has a normal range of development.

Some babies may skip stages. They may not crawl. They may go straight from rolling over to wanting to stand up and walk and never want to crawl. That's okay. It used to be felt that that was a missed stage of development and would lead to learning disabilities. Pediatricians and neurologists and so on do not believe that that is the case.

Steve: How about when they start laughing?

Dr. Bentley: Actually, laughter will occur somewhere between 2 and 4 months of age; when you start playing peek-a-boo with your baby or when you start tickling your baby. Some babies like their hips flexed or their feet stroked and they will break into broad laughter as early as 2 or 3 months of age.

Patti: When will they start speaking or trying to form words?

Dr. Bentley: The first developments are of course laughing, and then they will start cooing; making those kinds of sounds. Usually around 9 to 12 months of age you can pick out words that babies are saying. Extremely verbal babies will say intelligible words as early as 8 or 9 months of age. By a year of age we expect they will be saying 2 to 4 words. They will probably understand more than they will verbalize.

Now it is important to state that if a baby is not saying words at a year of age that is not a danger sign. This is so variable. It depends on a baby's personality, where they fit in the family. First babies are much more verbal than babies down the line. Every baby is different.

Patti: When would you ever be alarmed if some of these milestones didn't occur? Is there a rule of thumb?

Dr. Bentley: The rule of thumb is if a baby is missing several milestones then we become more concerned than if a baby misses an isolated milestone. For example, if a baby rolled over at 3 or 4 months was very socially interactive, smiled appropriately and so on but never crawled, I would never be concerned about that.

Patti: Okay.

Dr. Bentley: But if a baby didn't roll over until 9 or 10 months of age maybe, didn't crawl until 15 to 16 months of age, was not verbal, was not socially interactive, did not walk until well after 18 months of age, you know, there is a pattern there. This baby is way behind in every milestone and then you become very concerned.

Steve: Isn't it also important to talk to your baby? In other words I was aware of someone whose baby wasn't talking at the age of 3 or 4. They took the child and got him tested and found that there was absolutely nothing wrong but the parents never had spoken to the child.

Dr. Bentley: Yes.

Steve: And so the child didn't know what to do?

Dr. Bentley: Absolutely and that's one of the reasons why we believe firstborn children are more verbal and more interactive because parents do invest more time and energy into interacting with their baby. But yes, even from day one as you are nursing your baby, we believe you should talk to your baby and have eye contact. You know, there is that bonding that is important. It is not just this creature that you are going through the motions with. You should really interact. They are sponges that soak in more than you can imagine. Their environment teaches them incredible amounts every day of their life. Talk to them. Sing to them lullabies. Read to them, even though they are little tiny babies. That is what develops their language.

Steve: I was told to even tell them what you are doing.

Dr. Bentley: Sure.

Steve: If they are sitting in the crib and you are washing the dishes. Of course you wouldn't have the crib in the kitchen but–

Dr. Bentley: Or you might.

Steve: Tell them what you are doing.

Dr. Bentley: You might have a playpen in the kitchen with the baby right there.

Patti: Sure.

Dr. Bentley: There was an interesting study that came out of Harvard, that looked at very achieving children and the families of those children. I mean, very brilliant children. They were well above the norm in the country. And they looked at the families that these children or students came from and what was significant, or what was the common thread with these families. It was not upper crust families, it was not professional parents, it was not, you know, high class type people, it was all types of people, but the common thread was parents that interacted and talked to their children and babies. They wouldn't necessarily spend a lot of time with them. They would go about their chores. But they would take little moments that if a child showed some curiosity, maybe some interest in something, the mother just might bend down and spend a golden five seconds at that moment with that child and then go on with their chores.

CHAPTER TWENTY-FOUR

Umbilical Cord, Circumcision, Cleaning Genitalia

Steve: Dr. Bently what is your advice with regard to taking care of the baby's umbilical cord and circumcision.

Dr. Bentley: With regard to the umbilical cord I recommend using rubbing alcohol around the base of the cord about three times a day. If it's applied too much the cord really doesn't fall off within 1 to 2 weeks like it should. The umbilical cord actually rots through at the base and there is a lot of foul-smelling discharge, and that's normal. The application of the alcohol is just to keep that cleaned off so that it doesn't get infected. Cords normally are really foul smelling, and there's a lot of drainage especially as they're close to coming off. What you look for is if the cord is infected or not, the skin itself is real red and tender and hot and kind of hard around the base where the cord is. Whether or not there is foul-smelling discharge. But the rubbing alcohol should be applied about three times a day with a cotton ball or a clean washcloth.

You do not use soap on the umbilical cord, you do not use diaper wash or anything like that, just alcohol.

With regard to circumcision, there's two kinds of circumcisions. One is with a plastic ring called a plastibell, that normally comes off after about 5 to 7 days. And there's no particular care that needs to be delivered until the ring comes off. Once that comes off, or even partially comes off then you need to carefully clean around the new exposed area with each diaper change, particularly messy diapers, to make sure you get all the stool cleaned off.

Steve: Now cannot be done with the wipes, the diaper wipes.

Dr. Bentley: I recommend just water. The diaper wipes have too much alcohol in them, and that burns and stings and would be uncomfortable for the baby.

The other kind of circumcision is with a device called Gomco. The foreskin is taken completely off, and what you see is the finished product. The head of the penis is then real red and swollen for several days after that and has a coating, kind of a mucousy coating that looks like it might even be infected, especially if you're not used to seeing that.

The difference between an infected circumcision and a normal circumcision in that event is that the shaft of the penis is normal and not red and not tender. Whereas if it gets infected it really swells up and gets red and real tender below where the circumcision is. But the head of the penis and just below that usually gets real red and swollen in a normal circumcision. And again you just wipe around that with a clean cloth, a clean washcloth using clean water, usually tap water is fine, or a cotton ball and water, but not using any wipes or using any alcohol until it is fully healed up for at least a week. And that is with each diaper change. Then you can apply some Vaseline to the Gomco type circumcision, so that it doesn't adhere to the diaper and cause any discomfort or bleeding.

You might be interested with little girls how we would advise you to take care of their genital area. Often stool will get into the little crevices among the labia majora and labia minora and so we recommend very carefully, gently cleaning those areas.

There's a very tenacious, cheesy white kind of coating that's often present with little girls. Do not try to take that off because that will cause, you know, quite a bit of discomfort with a girl and if you try to rub that off, you'll actually cause sores and probably remove some of the skin in that area.

CHAPTER TWENTY-FIVE

Diaper Rash

Patti: How do you prevent diaper rash?

Dr. Bentley. That is a good question. You may not be able to prevent diaper rash. That is a loaded question. A lot of parents become very dismayed and upset when their babies get a diaper rash, because they're expectations are that if they are a good parent their baby will never have a diaper rash. But I am here to tell you that if your baby wears a diaper, they will have a diaper at some time during his life.

The best you can do is change your baby's diaper as frequently as possible, whenever it needs to be changed, and to have as good of hygiene as possible. But that is a very warm moist environment, and that is not good for skin, so therefore anytime you wear a diaper on your arm, on your leg, or in the diaper area, you will have a diaper rash. Thus, if you notice a diaper rash, you should take the baby's diaper off. It only makes sense, but parents will say, "What about my carpet?" You have to say, "Which is more important, my baby's diaper rash, or my carpet?" And the answer is that those of us that are seasoned parents will take our baby's diaper off, and either wrap a loose cloth type diaper on or a little towel or cloth, or if the baby is not even walking or crawling around, say just staying put as a one or two month old infant, who cares? Whether the baby's diaper is on or not you can just put the baby on a towel and you can wash the towel later. The more air that can get to the skin, the quicker the diaper rash will go away.

What then about all the diaper potions and lotions and creams and salves that you see on the market? Those are intended to guard the skin and protect the skin from the effects of stool, and urine and so on. The problem is, that is like wearing a raincoat in Florida in July, you get wetter inside from your sweat then you do from protecting your body from the rain. And if you put inclusive dressings like Desitin or A&D Ointment or whatever on a baby's diaper rash, you often are causing more harm than good. The best way to clear up a diaper rash is to actually let it air out, let it act like normal skin should act, and then put the diaper back on.

Patti: I have had some success trying to dry out a diaper rash with like a cornstarch powder. Does that make sense?

Dr. Bentley: Yes, cornstarch, or the powders made of cornstarch are very good at absorbing that extra moisture. So that does help. If you do use an ointment like, say you've aired out your baby's diaper area and you are ready to put the diaper back on. I like to use Vaseline. It is a lot lighter. It is easier to take off, it is not as tenacious, and it is protective, and still allows the skin to breathe some. That's my advice.

Steve: Dr. Bentley, are there some diaper rashes like yeast for example, that might need some special treatment in addition to what we've talked about for diaper rash?

Dr. Bentley: Yes, if a diaper rash does not improve with airing out or using the typical ointments and care that you have been instructed to use, if that does not clear up, then you should contact your pediatrician.

A yeast rash is typically in the creases in the groin area. And then it is very red and very weepy and at the edges of the rash, there are little red dots called satellite lesions. Yeast loves to grow in warm moist, dark environments. And so again if you wear a diaper, at some point you are going to have a yeast rash. Now, I know that some babies escape that, but the majority of babies will get a yeast rash, particularly if they go on antibiotics for an infection, they will often get a yeast rash. And that needs to be treated by special anti-yeast ointments that your doctor needs to prescribe.

Patti: I've heard that you can give your baby yogurt to help with that, does that make sense?

Dr. Bentley: It does make sense, and often that helps. If antibiotics kill good germs as well as bad germs, indiscriminately, and you are left without your normal population of bacteria that helps your body, then what happens is yeast comes in and grows where it normally wouldn't grow because your normal bacteria would keep it out. Just like a healthy lawn will keep out weeds. In a lawn that is not watered well or is not healthy, weeds will come in and grow. So, in an effort to repopulate your normal bacteria you can feed your baby yogurt and it will help.

Patti: At what age could you do that for an infant?

Dr. Bentley: Probably two or three months or older.

Steve: Now is that going against some advice about using dairy products and milk?

Dr. Bentley: We normally wouldn't feed yogurt as a food substance, except in this instance where maybe a baby has been on quite a bit of antibiotics and is having some yeast infections.

CHAPTER TWENTY-SIX

Car Seats

Steve: I think one of the first things that I remember, Dr Bentley, in leaving the hospital, is that the nurse, among other things, as she accompanied us out to the car, made sure we had a car seat.

Dr. Bentley: What a good nurse! It is sad when we invest so much effort in premature babies that are extremely ill, that may be in the hospital for several months and run up a bill of one or two million dollars, and then have them go home and not be in a car seat and get in a car accident. That unfortunately does happen.

One of the big mamers and injurers of children and babies is car accidents.

All babies should be in car seats period!

And there are car seats designed for infants, until they are toddlers. And then there are car seats designed for toddlers until they are older children, and then older children have booster seats. Obviously when they are old enough, they can sit in regular seats with seat belts.

Your pediatrician can help you with the brands and types and so on of car seats.

Suffice it to say that from birth until about 30 lbs, babies normally need to be facing the rear of the car, facing away from the front of the car and in car seats that have shoulder straps. And then from 30 lbs until about 45 to 50 lbs, they can be on booster seats. The reason for that is that the lap belt needs to go over the pelvis of a person. If a lap belt goes around the midsection, then it can lacerate or injure the liver or spleen. You don't want to be in an accident and have that belt hit a person in the midsection.

Younger children from 30 to 50 lbs need to be in a booster seat so that they can have the seat belt go over their pelvis instead of over their midsection. The additional advantage is that they can see outside better, and they like it better instead of down in the depths of a deeper seat.

Patti: I know some of the old car seats are not acceptable, so do you recommend going with a newer car seat?

Dr. Bentley: I do. The newer car seats abide by strict regulations, safety regulations. The top of the car seat needs to be anchored to the body frame of the car. The shoulder straps that go over the baby need to meet safety requirements so the baby can't wiggle out of them or squirt out of them in an accident. The body of the car seat needs to have certain requirements so that it doesn't crush. If the vehicle's seat folds during an accident, the car seat needs to withstand that pressure, so it won't fold. With many of the older car seats, the armrest was flimsy and would act as a weapon and club the baby over the head, etc.

There are many changes that have occurred in car seats. And again, there are a lot of different kinds of car seats and any given car may accommodate a certain style of car seat better. So which car seat you buy depends on the age and size of your child and the type of car you have.

If you do not have a car seat or cannot afford one, then you need to check around and find out about the availability of car seats. Because there are a lot of people and agencies that feel strongly about that and will make that available for you.

I feel that it is very important that babies, from the very start, know what it is like to sit in car seats and get used to it. They should never know what it is like to sit in the car without a car seat. Parents often think that they can nurse their babies while they are riding in the car, or hold the baby because they are strong enough to hold their baby safely. They think that if they are ever in an accident they will be able to keep their child from harm. That is absolutely wrong! The forces in an accident are incredible.

At 20 to 30 miles an hour, which would be the typical accident that occurs on your neighborhood streets, the forces are so incredible, that there is not a person alive that is strong enough to hold a baby from crashing into a windshield or the dashboard of a car.

Patti: It is also, from what I understand, a mistake to think that you can buckle them in with you.

Dr. Bentley: You will have a squashed child.

Steve: Dr. Bentley, what is your advice for childproofing your home?

Dr. Bentley: I think that part of having a child is making sure your baby, when he or she becomes mobile, cannot get into your cleaning supplies or anything else that is potentially dangerous. One of the favorite places for babies obviously, is the pot and pan drawer. That is even better than any Fisher-Price toy that you could ever buy a child. However, cupboards, where cleaning supplies are kept, need to have child safety locks. And there are a lot of child-proof locks that can be installed, such that you can get in but the child cannot. There are little nylon locks that snap closed when the door is closed, and don't require a key or anything. Those cupboards and drawers all need to be locked, especially if they hold sharp implements, knives, etc. Any type of cupboards or drawers that hold medications or chemicals need to be locked.

When your child becomes mobile, it's not too long before your child will start climbing. And then any cabinet and every cabinet is fair game. I often have parents say, "But, but, I didn't think my child could reach that cabinet at six months of age!" And it totally flabbergasted them when they came into a room and found their child in the middle of a bottle of pills. So as long as you are childproofing the lower cabinets, you may as well childproof all cabinets that have any kind of dangerous items.

CHAPTER TWENTY-SEVEN

Baby Swings and Walkers

Patti: I've heard some concerns about using baby walkers. What's your advice?

Dr. Bentley: Baby walkers can be wonderful things to entertain your toddler. When the baby is around six or seven months of age, that can be a very grumpy time for them. They want to get around, but yet they can't quite be as mobile as they would like. So having swings, having jumpers, having walkers, are great little items, however they are very very dangerous. You have to be particularly careful where stairways are exposed for them to go crashing down the stairway.

If you have a walker-- and I don't advise against a walker, but I do advise that you are very cautious about figuring out where a baby can get into trouble. For example, the hearth of a fireplace. They can bump into that and sustain a laceration of the forehead. For sure, all stairways need to have childproof gates installed. And you say, "Well ,that marks up my wall!" Well, that's too bad. That's the price you pay for having a toddler. And then you can just redo it and fill in the holes when your child grows up. But you do need to have some gates to go across stairways and to protect any pitfall, if you will, where they can fall down. And then you need to supervise. You can't just walk out of the room and expect that your child is going to be perfectly safe. That is when accidents happen. You really need to supervise your child at all times.

Steve: You talked about having those gates permanently installed. I've seen some that, I don't know if it is by spring or something, but you can just place them there and they move around pretty easily. Do you recommend against those?

Dr. Bentley: I do, because those little accordion gates can pinch babies little fingers and hands. In fact, fingers can actually get cut off. And without very much pushing, those gates will come down and they will go crashing down the stairways. I've seen a lot of accidents from those.

CHAPTER TWENTY-EIGHT

Choking

Patti: Dr. Bentley, what foods should we avoid giving our baby?

Dr. Bentley: There are some really famous choking foods that are available for babies, particularly popcorn, peanuts, anything that is small and round and that they will try to swallow without chewing.

A good rule of thumb is that anytime you put your baby in a highchair, and put food on the tray, you need to be available. You need to be supervising that even if you are cooking dinner or on the phone or doing other chores, you need to be watchful of that baby. Anything you give your baby can potentially be choked on.

Popcorn peanuts, little peas come especially frozen peas, anything like that, our little easy objects for a baby to choke on. I recommend strongly against popcorn and peanuts. I think peas are an okay item to give, but again with good watchful supervision.

Steve: How about that zwieback toast? We gave our child that, and he really enjoyed it, but then it started to get soggy, and before you know it he had a pretty good chunk in his mouth that we had to fish out real quick because we thought he was going to choke on it.

Dr. Bentley: The value of zwieback and arrowroot teething type biscuits or cookies is that they are designed for the toddler and they become soggy and gooey, rather than fragments off like a saltine cracker. Saltines and graham crackers are a little more dangerous than the teething biscuits and cookies and you can fish that out of his mouth, before he chokes on it. That's the beauty of being available and supervising and knowing what's going on, otherwise he could have choked. And it only takes seconds, when a baby is choking, maybe a minute, to a minute and a half before they are unconscious without air.

Patti: Dr. Bentley, what do we do if we find that our child is choking?

Dr. Bentley: I think every parent should be knowledgeable with the Heimlich maneuver, with adults and with children. Children are very easy to manipulate, they are small you can pick them up, if you put the doubled-up fist in the pit of their stomach and their back is facing your chest, and then with your doubled up fist in the pit of their stomach you forcefully pull in, that should pop out anything that is trapped in their mouth or throat. It is recommended that you first try to fish out anything in their mouths, but not too aggressively, because you can lodge something further in if you're not too careful.

I think it is wise that every parent takes a CPR course that is offered in any of the neighboring hospitals, particularly children's hospitals in your area, to learn such skills.

Steve: Does a person need to be a little more cautious with an infant or a child than with an adult? Say a child is choking versus an adult choking on a piece of meat or something.

Dr. Bentley: Well the same caution applies, but obviously adults can handle their own affairs easier than infants. Infants and young children are totally dependent on adults, their parents. You need to be sure that your fist isn't over the rib cage. It needs to be right in the pit of the stomach, the soft part of the stomach, not too low. It needs to be above the navel and below the rib cage or you will break some ribs or maybe lacerate one of the organs in the abdomen.

Patti: I know that I have been instructed to pound on their back.

Dr. Bentley: That is also part of it. If someone is choking, you try to dislodge it by pounding on their back, you strike two or three times on their back, and you do a mouth sweep, but some people are even advising against that because you can force it further down if you don't dislodge it with the pounding on the back, then you do the Heimlich maneuver.

Steve: What about swallowing objects, swallowing a coin, or really anything a child can get his or her hands on?

Dr. Bentley: That is a concern. It is incredible what kids can swallow. They will swallow anything that is pointed and dangerous and sharp. Usually things like that, incredibly enough, will pass.

I had a patient once who swallowed a full-size, brand new, number 2 pencil with a sharp point on it. And when I called the surgeon, he said don't worry about it. It will pass. We took an x-ray and we watched and a day or two later it came through.

Coins are a concern, pennies, dimes, nickels, because they can get lodged in a little pocket at the junction of where the esophagus joins onto the stomach. They can lodge there and then they can erode through the wall of the esophagus and stomach. That can lead to death. So therefore, any child who swallows a coin should be checked out by a physician. Usually we will take an x-ray to see where the coin is and if it is past that little anatomical juncture point, then a child should be fine. The coin will pass. Things like little batteries to watches are a real concern because they can dissolve and the mercury in them will be really dangerous.

Occasionally other sharp objects need to be fished out. Anything you have a concern for like this, you need to call your doctor and check it out.

Patti: Sometimes children will push objects in their ears or up their nose, what do you do if you have found that has happened?

Dr. Bentley: Well if you can get it out easily enough at home that is fine, otherwise we can fish it out at the office. I don't recommend punishing the child. "Let's take him into the doctors and punish him by having the doctor make it real painful."

We get those objects out pretty easily with our instruments and try to make it as painless as possible. Children normally like to put things into their ears and noses and you just do your best to teach them not to but it is just part of childhood for them to to do that.

Like almost any childhood behavior, the more attention you draw to that, the more the child will often be attracted to that behavior. If you are all upset and nervous and on your high horse when a child puts their finger in their nose, I can assure you that that will be something they will try to repeat and enhance on.

CHAPTER TWENTY-NINE

Swallowing Poison

Patti: What should we do if our child takes in poison?

Doctor Bentley: As much as you try to protect your child from dangerous chemicals and cleaning supplies and medications and so on, the chance exists that your child will get into something like that. The best advice will be to either call your pediatrician, or if your community has a poison control or poison information center, you can call them. Some poisons or strong chemicals burn and scar on the way down and so we don't want to induce vomiting because they will burn on the way up. And that's the whole reason behind not sometimes inducing vomiting.

Usually the advice is that ipecac, the chemical that is available to purchase from pharmacies, is kept in your medicine cabinet. You can give that to your kids when they have swallowed something that you need to get out. Now you give that upon the advice of the Poison Control Center or your physician. And include plenty of water and then if vomiting does not occur, then that child should be rushed to the emergency room or, in the event that enough has been swallowed that it is a dangerous amount, that you give ipecac and then you had to the emergency room expecting that the child will throw up on the way. That way, you have bought some time before you get to the emergency room and then other measures will be taken.

Steve: Do you ever use an ipecac if you swallow something, like if they swallow a coin? If you're worried about it, do you give them ipecac?

Dr. Bentley: We never use ipecac for swallowed objects. It seems way too severe to cause a child to retch and vomit repeatedly for something that will usually pass on its own. Plus, you usually cannot make an object go back up once it is down. It needs to be retrieved if it's in the wrong place.

Steve: And how is that retrieval done, through surgery?

Dr. Bentley: Through scoping. Usually the child needs to be anesthetized. The physician will go down through the esophagus and grab it with a little grasp, trap device and pull it back out.

Steve: What does it mean when a hospital pumps the child's

stomach?

Dr. Bentley: That means that there is still enough poison in the stomach, and the stomach's bowels, that they try to wash out the stomach and retrieve as much as they can. It's called lavaging. They put down a big bore catheter into the stomach and they pump saltwater into the stomach and they suck it back out, retrieving as much of the chemical or pill fragments as they can. Because a lot of the poison will have already passed into the small bowel and they can't get it out through pumping the stomach, then they put in activated charcoal in a slurry, which then goes down and absorbs all of that poison and does not allow it to be absorbed into the body.

CHAPTER THIRTY

Medicines and Immunizations

Patti: Dr. Bentley, what should we have in our medicine chest for our baby?

Dr. Bentley: A really good kit for your baby medication wise, would be a fever reducer, acetaminophen, a common brand name would be Tylenol or Tempra, or any of the generic brands of acetaminophen are just as fine.

Ibuprofen comes in a liquid and is available by prescription through your Physician's office and is very good for reducing fever. One that used to be used a lot was baby aspirin, however that is not recommended anymore for reduction of fever when children are sick or even for use of pain. The reason being that it has clearly been associated with a severe illness called Reye's syndrome that attacks a baby's or a child's liver and carries a 50% mortality rate. It is clearly associated with the use of aspirin when children are sick.

Steve: How common is Reye's syndrome?

Dr Bentley: It is quite rare, but when it happens it is very severe and lethal.

Usually, most medicine cabinets will have a decongestant that you might give your baby or child for a cold and a cough. And I would consult your Physician's office for their recommended brands and dosages. Those are usually age-appropriate and size appropriate dosages.

You should have something for diarrhea, which we do not recommend you use unless you have consulted your position. There are some good over-the-counter anti-diarrheal liquids, but you should consult your physician first.

Patti: Do you recommend using the gels?

Doctor Bentley: For teething?

Patti: Yes.

Dr. Bentley: Those are often helpful anesthetics to put on baby's gums when they are teething for temporary relief. Likewise there are anesthetic sprays and gels for sunburns, mosquito bites, rashes, that can be purchased and some are quite good.

Of course, sunblocks and sunscreens, anything you can do to

prevent injury is recommended over something to treat it after it has already happened.

Steve: We've talked a little bit about check-ups and well-baby visits. Can you tell us a little bit about immunizations and how important they are?

Dr. Bentley: Immunizations have done more to help us raise our children in good health than almost anything else. Perhaps antibiotics would be in that same category.

If you think about families that would lose half of their children to diphtheria or polio or whooping cough, we don't see those diseases anymore. And that is because of immunizations. And unless we all take a very small risk with our children of an occasional fever or perhaps even more seriously, and occasional seizure or convulsion with some of these immunizations, there will be many children who won't be immunized and there will be an un-immunized population that will continue these horrible childhood illnesses. For example, in the eastern United States among the Amish people who don't believe in modern medicine and advances, polio still occurs with their children.

Sometimes among people that immigrated to the United States we see childhood diseases that we rarely see in our own children, for example, measles. So I cannot stress enough that if you don't do anything else with your children, but get their immunizations, you'll be much farther ahead than our ancestors were just 100 years ago.

This concludes the presentation of
Let's Talk Babies

featuring
Dr. L. Frank Bentley

answering questions
from parents Patti and Steve

A Note from the Editor

As editor, I would like to give special thanks and credit to Mark Dixon and Rudy Taylor, the producers of the original recording made at CDI Studios.

It's hard to believe that these timeless productions all started when they first asked me to record a project titled: The Proper Care of Ferrets as Pets.

Thanks Mark and Rudy for your mature guidance and friendship over the years.

This presentation is also available as an eBook and the original Audiobook format.

Published by Walkercrest copyright 2021